Preface

This is the back story, that helps you begin to understand, the journey I will be taking you on. I was born on a cold winter morning in 1965. LOL. No, no, no, we are definitely not going that far back. Trust me when I say I have done all I can to streamline this information so that it is most beneficial to you the reader.

Prior to all this 2010: My wife was diagnosed with stage 4 terminal lung cancer, and I became her caretaker. We have 5 kids, 3 still living at home at the time. I was working (driving) at a trucking company, working nights, 12-14-hour workdays. During the day I took care of my wife and took her to doctor appointments, etc., I barely slept well at all. My wife's health deteriorated horribly through the years. It was beginning to take its toll on me.

August 2014: I had a stroke, collapsed, blacked out, no feeling or even ability to use my left side at all. Rushed to the hospital. Hospital misdiagnosed me, after being there all day, then they sent me home. Two days later, I was experiencing speech and comprehension issued, called my doctor immediately. They said, "Jim, you are having a stroke get to the hospital immediately." They sent me to another hospital that specialized in neurology. There they kept me and diagnosed my situation and made me aware that I had two strokes and that there are scares on my brain from them. Two weeks out of work and I went back to work and back to the same grindstone of schedule and responsibility.

March 2015: After blacking out two times in the warehouse I went to see my neurologist. He hospitalized me for 3 ½ weeks and took me out of work permanently and put me on 3 stroke medications.

November 26, 2016: My wife passed away. It took till 2018 for me to do what you are about to read. And now my life is much different and I got my health back.

CONTENTS

My Journey to Serious Weight Loss

This is my story.

Introduction

The blunt of this book has been written by me as this progress and transformation occurred in real time. This is more or less a diary, written by me and edited by me.

This is my story.

This is now the following year and I am came back to this diary and filled in all the details of so much that I did to accomplish this incredible transformation. It is raw and at times mundane, but please know, this worked for me. Maybe a variation of this will work for you.

Keto works! The thing I learned is that you must make it work for you, not you conform to it. In other words, build the depths of your own personal research into it and then from it, build it around your life, your likes and dislikes and what works best for you.

You'll see by my food choices, the way I cooked them and how I combined them, that I did Keto my way. I have often referred to this as my Keto Mojo... For me that means Keto (**M**y **O**wn **J**immy **O**utcome) Mojo. Through my own research, I learned how to know why I want better higher quality nutrients in my diet instead of the cheapest foods I can buy. I also learned so much about the benefits of Intermittent Fasting and fasting in general. Keep studying and researching, other then your doctors, who knows your body better then you? No one. So, you will know what will work and what you wouldn't mind doing.

When I was asked what are you doing? I typically would say, "In many ways I have become my own personal nutritionist." Keep that in mind as you consider to really focus on losing weight and becoming healthy.

Chapter 1

My Journey Has Begun

Sunday of the morning, of the day I began, I weighed in at 271lbs. This is a picture of me with some friends having lunch in an Italian Restaurant, the week prior to this weigh in. My downfall has always been food and soda (*the dew and cream soda*). You see, I love food, I crave it. And honestly some days I can never get enough. I still desire and crave foods, but not like before.

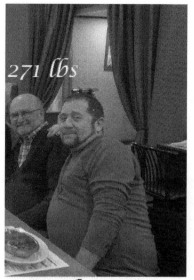

271 lbs

Early 2018

This was a pretty horrifying reality of what I used to look like. In July I went to Arizona to see my son and his wife, but mostly to go see my grandson. On that trip, I ate wiser and I walked an hour every single day. Early mornings in Arizona are very beautiful.

After seeing my weight drop so much from my 2-weeks in Arizona, I was inspired to start working on losing weight. But, upon my return home, I simply went back to my old habits and my weight sky-rocketed once again. I know that I really need to make serious changes in my life, and they need to be ones that will inevitably be my lifestyle, not simply a diet. I really didn't just want to go on some diet.

There are so many foods I will always want to eat, so how do I do this. Simple: I began researching online, what could possibly be a good, healthy alternative to improve my health. I even consulted my doctors explaining my intentions, they offered help and assistance when I needed it, especially along the way. After all my doctors know my health situation best and all the medication I was taking.

In the past I have fasted for many reasons. What I have noticed from all those years of fasting for a day here and there and even an occasional 5-day fast; was that my health, my skin and my body felt so refreshed and as an added bonus, I even lost weight. But then of cause I returned to my old habits. So, nothing was really changing, or gained and in the end, the benefits I was gaining weren't lasting.

Days 1 and 2 of this journey you are reading about, were experimental. I'm just saying those 2 days, I did fast, and I did eat, but I was just learning. Here is exactly what I did.

Chapter 2

I Officially Began on Day 3

I officially began on the 3rd day to Intermittently Fast at a 23:1 ratio. I said to myself, if I am going to do this, I am all in and I am looking for a dramatic serious change in my life. The 23:1 means, that I fast for 23 hours and then there is an open window of 1 hour to eat. I have learned a lot in the past few days on what is the best and the healthiest way to do this.

Each day's meal had 2 goals:
Calories (*for energy*) and
Nutrition (*for optimum health*).

Today has been a very exciting day, my first real official taste, no pun intended, of what I am about to undertake, and you want to know something? I am not even hungry. In the morning I only drink one bottle of water (16.9 oz.) so I can take my vitamins and my meds. Just to let you know, I take 3 blood pressure pills and 1 cholesterol pill, plus I take 2 other medications for my stroke side effects. So, there is a lot going on when I began this. Hence, why I made sure my doctors knew what was going on. Every morning I will dry fast, meaning no water till I eat. My dry fast actually begins when I fall asleep the night before.

Here is something else I learned about Intermittent Fasting. This type of fasting maximizes your Growth Hormone which is the main fat burning hormone and the main hormone for lean body mass. And as an added bonus, it is an anti-aging hormone as well. There are tremendous benefits to fasting, especially intermittent fasting. See, with intermittent fasting, you get to eat, and you get to rest your body. Unlike regular fasting involving no intake of food, you will eventually return to eating again and that could change the results. This form of fasting helps you to develop healthier eating habits.

Here is my day:

Woke up at 3:30am. (*by choice*)
In the morning I am most productive, I have prayer and writing/research time, so by choice I wake up super early and begin my day. Today, after letting my dog out I got a bottle of water and I added a teaspoon of *Apple Cider Vinegar* to it. That is what I drank while taking my vitamins and my medication. I really hope to get off these pills soon, once I really begin to get my healthy life back. You will see this is how I start every day, seven days a week, even when I go away. Here is my day.

- 6:15- 7:00 a.m. (*I walked approximately 1.6 miles*)
- 9:05- 10:00 a.m. (*I took a second walk of 2.0 miles*)
Total miles walked today: 3.6

Waking is my exercise of choice for now. I find it very relaxing and it's not stressful on my body right now. I get to breath in the fresh air and I get to walk through town and see many of my friends as I am walking. So, in my eye I see it as a great health benefit both physically and emotionally. I am widower and so using a treadmill would not benefit me in so many ways. I need to get out and about and see other people. I am in such a better place today, since walking is part of this whole transformation of my life. Maybe in my next book I will write all about the true lasting benefits of walking.

If you feel led to do this, you should first consult your doctor. My doctor is well aware of what I am doing, and he said I can email him or call him if I have any questions. I believe you to should do the same. Everyone's health is unique and different to the needs and issues we all face. Please be safe. Since I had 2 strokes in 2014, walking when I was able to, was truly the only exercise I could do.

This was my 1 and only meal today: (12 noon to 12:35 p.m.)

½ Pint of fresh Blueberries (110 calories)
2 slices of Swiss Cheese (212 calories)
1.5 pounds of Chicken that I boiled in water (750 calories)
2 cups of Sweet Potato Fries, baked (344 calories)
1 small Vanilla Ice Cream Sandwich (160 calories)
And a bottle of Water (16.9 oz.)

My total calorie intake today is: 1,576

I looked online what my body needs daily, and this is what I have found:
To maintain my weight of 271, my BMR is 3,031 calories every day.
To lose weight they suggest, I need 2,241 calories every day.
To lose weight at an accelerated rate, I need 1,949 calories or less every day.

Just to let you know, you DO NOT have to calorie count once you get the knack of putting together a healthy meal that satisfies your days calorie intake, so you have energy. I chose to count calories, so I can teach myself how to put together a really healthy meal; one that would make me feel full, not bloated, just contently full. This is not intended to be a fast with no food. So, we have to utilize the eating time, to get in our days food. In the long run I can see how exciting and fun and healthy this will be to have a schedule of 7 healthy meals a week.

Then at 1:30 p.m. – Bottle of Water (16.9 oz.) *I add lemon to all my water.*

Also, at 2:30, 4:40 and then 6:20 p.m. – Bottle of Water (16.9 oz. each)

Total water today was: 84.5 oz. I think I need to raise that number

I was asleep by 8:30 p.m.

Chapter 3

I Am Starting To Feel More Energy

This is Day #4 of this journey. I read about energy levels increasing and honestly, today I feel the difference in how much more energy I have. And mind you I haven't even eaten anything since 12:30 p.m. yesterday. In the past I would feel sluggish and worn down, not today or any of these past few days. I feel an explosion of energy running through my body and it feels great.

Here is my day:

Woke up at 3:30am. (*by choice*)
In the morning I am most productive, I have prayer time and writing/research time, so by choice I wake up super early and begin my day. Today, the same as yesterday, after letting my dog out I got a bottle of water and I added a teaspoon

of *Apple Cider Vinegar* to it. That is what I drank while taking my vitamins and my medication. See how I start every day, seven days a week.
Here is my day.

- 6:20- 7:05 a.m. (*I walked approximately 1.5 miles*)
- 9:00- 9:50 a.m. (*I took a second walk of 1.8 miles*)
Total miles walked today: 3.3

As a side note, scattered whenever I feel an urge to eat something, I simple eat a fresh clove of garlic. Each clove is only 4 calories. Garlic Cloves have many benefits including: helping you maintain blood pressure and blood sugar levels, it can boost your immune system and so much more. I recommend you look into it, some of us can handle while others can't.

This was my 1 and only meal today: (11:30 – 11:55 a.m.)
From 11:15 a.m. till 11:30 I was cooking and preparing.

1 Pint of fresh Blueberries (220 calories)
8 oz. of Boneless/Skinless Salmon -baked (440 calories)
2 cups of vegetables -corn/peas (255 calories)
2 cups of Sweet Potato Fries, baked (344 calories)
2 small Vanilla Ice Cream Sandwich (320 calories)
And a bottle of Water.

My total calorie intake today is: 1,579

Wow, oddly enough my calorie count today was almost the same as yesterday's. I didn't plan the numbers that way, but I did want to plan a different variety, and I seem to have a much more sweeter tooth today. That is why I had 2 Ice Cream sandwiches.

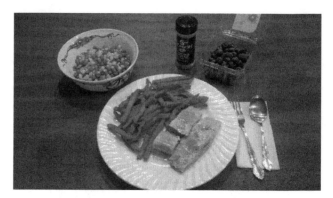

Day #4 Meal – Salmon on Sweet Potato Sticks

This afternoon I have been doing some online research and some laundry; through it all I felt very energetic and I'm surprisingly not hungry at all.

Then at 1:00 p.m. – Bottle of Water (16.9 oz.)

Also, at 2:15, 3:35, 4:30 and then 6:30 p.m. – Bottle of Water (16.9 oz. each)

Total water today was: 101.4 oz. I like that amount better. Staying hydrated is so important during this experience of intermittent fasting. That was my doctor's advice as I began this journey

I was asleep by 9:30 p.m.

Chapter 4

It's Starting To Feel Good

It is really amazing how good I am feeling on Day #5. My body is resting more throughout the day; and my digestive system isn't getting all kinds of snacks throughout the day, like I use to eat. My eating habits are beginning to tame down a lot and I am not even hungry, that's the best part. I feel content. I feel so much more energetic; I don't feel that bloated feeling of being full anymore. And honestly my t-shirt feels so much looser now (size 2x). I can feel that I am losing weight this week. Before I began this journey, size 2x was getting to be tight on me.

Here is my day:

Woke up at 3:45am. (*by choice*)
In the morning I am most productive, I have prayer time and writing/research time, so by choice I wake up super early and begin my day. Today, the same as yesterday (most everyday), after letting my dog out I got a bottle of water and I added a teaspoon of *Apple Cider Vinegar* to it.

My morning walks:

- 6:10- 6:55 a.m. (*I walked approximately 1.6 miles*)
- 8:50- 9:55 a.m. (*I took a second walk of 2.0 miles*)
Total miles walked today: 3.6

Today I woke up feeling really good. It's not that I don't feel good, but overall because of my stroke side effects; and my left side always being numb, for the most part, so I don't. It must be the changes in my eating habits and the fact that I am walking twice a day that rest is beginning to feel like rest.

This was my 1 and only meal today: (12:15 – 12:55 p.m.)
I started cooking and preparing at noon.

½ Pint of fresh Blueberries (110 calories)
1 lb. of Chicken Tenderloins, boiled in water (440 calories)
        (boneless and skinless)
2 cups of vegetables -corn/peas (255 calories)
1 Large fresh Sweet Potato (114 calories)

And a bottle of Water.

My total calorie intake today is: 919

I know that calorie count seems low, but I will say that was a lot to eat and I ate it all. It's been a good day, I don't feel the sense of hunger at all going all these hours without food. In-fact it seems like the opposite, at least for me. Once my stomach is filled and I get busy with my writing projects or other hobbies I have, I am totally distracted, and hunger don't even enter my thoughts.

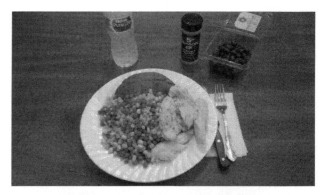

Day #5 Meal – Chicken Potato Vege Pile

This afternoon I have been writing and doing some house cleaning. Today I am working on reorganizing the Family Room, where we store some stuff, but through it all, I am not hungry at all.

Then at 1:30 p.m. – Bottle of Water (16.9 oz.)

Also, at 2:40, 3:45, 4:55 and then 6:20 p.m. – Bottle of Water (16.9 oz. each)

Total water today was: 101.4 oz. (same as yesterday) This should be norm, staying hydrated is so important during intermittent fasting.

I was asleep by 8:15 p.m.

Chapter 5

Progress Is Beginning To Happen

Day #6: I am amazed, but not surprised. I will say that I am noticing a huge change in my sleep. I feel much more rested lately. In the past, well, just prior to all this, I can sleep 4-6 hours a night and feel perfectly well. Yes, but truth be known, by 5-6 p.m. I would feel sluggish and; even though this early morning wake-up is my routine, there are many mornings I have to push myself through those early hours. Now with this new pattern of eating and my 2 walks in the morning, sleep is easy now, and I do want a little more. I seem to be averaging about 7 hours now and it feels great.

Here is my day:

Woke up at 3:15am. (*by choice*)
In the morning I am most productive, I have prayer time and writing/research time, so by choice I wake up super early and begin my day. Today, the same as yesterday (most everyday), after letting my dog out I got a bottle of water and I added a lemon to my water this morning. I don't know why I just did.

My morning walks:

- 6:05- 6:45 a.m. (*I walked approximately 1.8 miles*)
- 7:00- 7:55 a.m. (*I took a second walk of 1.9 miles to Key Foods*)
- 9:30- 10:05 a.m. (*I even took a third walk I am so filled with energy 2.0 miles*)
Total miles walked today: 5.7

Today I woke up feeling the best ever in a long time. It absolutely must be the changes in my eating habits and all these hours of fasting. I have also learned that

Ketosis kicks in at about 4th or 5th day and it has been said in so many places that I researched; our bodies become fat burning machines. I feel some major boost of energy and it really feels good. Today I feel like eating a huge salad with some chicken on top.

This was my 1 and only meal today: (11:55 a.m. to 12:25 p.m.)
I precooked the chicken early in the morning, so it can cool down.

½ Pint of fresh Blueberries (110 calories)
12 oz. of mixed Salad -Dole bag (60 calories)
6 oz. Mandarin Oranges (100 calories)
1.3 lb. of Chicken Breast, boiled in water (586 calories)
        (boneless and skinless chicken from Perdue)
1 fresh Avocado (234 calories)
And a bottle of water.

My total calorie intake today is: 1,090

Yes indeed, this is a bit of a different meal than the last few, I like variety and I really like salads. There is a of chicken in that salad and this is a huge bowl. It felt so good eating this today.

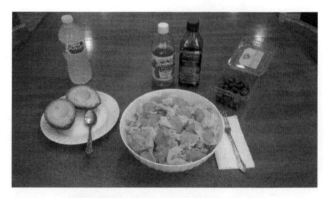

Day #6 Meal – Chicken Salad Citrus

This afternoon is just one of those rare days that I am overflowing with so much energy. Today I am going through my Baseball Card collection, to organize and hopefully sell. Yes, it's not a physical task, but with that said; sometimes those tasks with minimal energy become very exhausting. I am not tired at all, I still feel like I am overflowing with so much energy.

Then at 1:15 p.m. – Bottle of Water (16.9 oz.)

Also, at 2:30, 3:50, 5:05 and then 6:10 p.m. – Bottle of Water (16.9 oz. each)

Total water today was: 101.4 oz. (same as yesterday) Like I said before, this should be my norm, staying hydrated is so important during intermittent fasting. It's actually important no matter what you are doing.

I was asleep by 8:00 p.m.

Chapter 6

The Energy Is Now Overflowing

Day #7: This has really been a very beneficial journey for me. I can already feel so many of my eating habits being broken. No, my eating habits weren't always healthy. They were healthier prior to Chrissy's illness and then my strokes. But now, I can see and sense that I am moving in the right direction. Last night my son Travis brought home a box of Chinese food, I love that stuff. Normally, he would say, or I would ask and before you know I would be eating it for hours. But, no, not last night, I was able to just walk by, knowing that I am really not hungry anyway and it didn't faze me.

Here is my day:

Woke up at 3:00am. (*by choice*)
I just ended up falling asleep so early last night, so by 3 a.m. I looked at the clock and I knew I couldn't just lay here anymore. I woke up very energetic again. I did my usual routine, put my dog outside, got my bottle of water and I began my routine with prayer and writing.

My morning walks:

- 5:50- 7:30 a.m. (*I walked 3.5 miles, even with the numbness in my left leg*)
- 8:30- 9:25 a.m. (*I just took this walk, 2 laps around town, 2.2 miles*)
- 9:55- 10:45 a.m. (*I just couldn't resist another walk around town, 1.6 mile*)
Total miles walked today: 7.3 (*ambitious day*)

Today I woke up feeling just as much energy as yesterday, if not even more. There is no doubt that Ketosis has kicked in; I am feeling lighter, more refreshed and even with 7 hours sleep I feel amazing. Tomorrow is Weigh In day, I will be surprised by any huge weight loss, I really can feel a huge different in my body.

This was my 1 and only meal today: (12:00 p.m. to 12:30 p.m.)
It was a simple meal to prepare, I cooked everything at the same time.

5 Scrambled Eggs, fried (450 calories)
4 Sausage Links, fried (200 calories)
4.5 oz. of French Fries, microwaved (100 calories)
2 tablespoons of Maple Syrup (104 calories)
1 fresh Avocado (234 calories)
And a bottle of water.

My total calorie intake today is: 1,178

It was "Big Breakfast" my one meal a day time for me. I was just experimenting, putting together a nice size breakfast that would fill me. I can't image the way I use it eat. This could have been a typical breakfast, not counting snacks, and other meals. I feel content and I feel so much healthier.

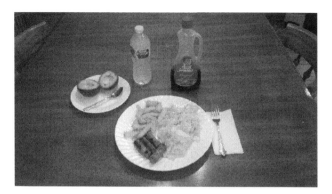

Day #7 Meal – Big Breakfast Avocado

This afternoon I have been writing and doing some house cleaning. Today I am working on reorganizing the basement more, but through it I am not hungry at all.

Then at 1:00 p.m. – Bottle of Water (16.9 oz.)

Also, at 2:05, 3:30, 4:25 and then 6:00 p.m. – Bottle of Water (16.9 oz. each)

Total water today was: 101.4 oz. (same as yesterday) This continues to be my norm, staying hydrated is so important every single day even if you are not fasting. Repetitive yes, but very important.

I was asleep by 7:30 p.m.

Chapter 7

My First Weeks Results

I know it is Day #8. But since I started on Sunday, those will be my Weigh In Days. This is my first full week of very dedicated Intermittent Fasting with 23 hour a day fast and I am easting only one meal. This is called the OMAD diet. I don't know why they call it diet, because it is more like a lifestyle. I lost 22 pounds. I know that sounds crazy, but I am fat, I admit that. But I also know that every week won't be like this. This is my first week of dramatic change in years.

Wow!! How about them apples! LOL !!! Nice weight loss in one week. This OMAD Lifestyle is new to me, but I really like it and I am further encouraged when I see such results. And to think I didn't join a club or have to buy special foods. I simple watched what I ate and made sure I walked each day. Though I have read most people that lost a lot of weight doing this, didn't really focus on any specific exercise regimen.

Here is my day:

Woke up at 3:20 am. (*hearing heavy thundershowers this morning*)
I ended up falling asleep so early last night, so by 3 a.m. I was awake. Yesterday, I did a lot of walking and it felt great, so did my sleep. This morning I woke up very energetic again. I did my usual routine, put my dog outside, got my bottle of water and I began my routine with prayer and writing.

My morning walks: (*the rain today won't stop me*)

- 7:00- 7:45 a.m. (*I walked in the rain, it felt amazing for 1.2 miles*)
- 10:00- 10:15 a.m. (I walked but my left leg let out because it's numb, time for
        me rethink all this walking, it maybe too much on my stroke side-effects.)
Total miles walked today: 1.2

Today I woke up feeling so much more energy. I think this is becoming my new norm. I used to feel so tired and run down from doing nothing. I hated that, but I knew it was diet and my physical shape that caused it. I am so grateful that I have finally got the excitement too make this optimum health happen in my life again. Just remember, this is my story.

But now after I did all this walking these past few days, I am honestly starting to feel the pain in my left side even more. Like I said in earlier chapters, I had 2 strokes in 2014 that left my left side completely numb. I think I have just been taking for granite, that I can do it, I really need to be careful. Full stop on my walks for now. My doctors even said, pull back on the walking for now. I need to recover from this, but I am not stopping this new OMAD Lifestyle. My numbness is on my left side, shoulder to my toes. Right now I am stopping all walking, lets see how this lifestyle alone can cut the pounds.

This was my 1 and only meal today: (12:00 p.m. to 12:35 p.m.)

½ pint of fresh Blueberries (110 calories)
4 oz. Wild Caught Salmon, microwaved (440 calories)
6 oz. of Mandarin Oranges (100 calories)
1 Sweet Potato, microwaved (110 calories)
19 oz of Broccoli Cuts, microwaved (100 calories)
1 fresh Avocado (234 calories)
And a bottle of water.

My total calorie intake today is: 1,094

Today I looked at what was left in the house, so I can assemble a meal. I am not too thrilled to have a mostly microwaved meal, but both the sweet potato and the broccoli are packaged in such a way that they can be microwaved. And the Salmon cooks easily in the microwave. Things will change as time moves on and I have a handle on healthier way to prepare my meal each day.

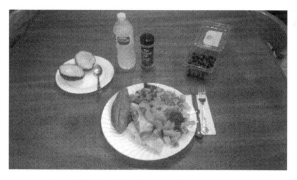

Day #8 Meal - Leftovers Extravaganza

This afternoon I have been writing and doing some house cleaning. Today I am working in the basement going through more stuff.

Then at 1:20 p.m. – Bottle of Water (16.9 oz.)

Also, at 2:30, 3:40, 4:15 and then 5:50 p.m. – Bottle of Water (16.9 oz. each)

Total water today was: 101.4 oz. (same as yesterday) This again continues to be my norm, staying hydrated is so important every single day even if you are not fasting.

I was asleep by 8:00 p.m.

Chapter 8

Blah... Blah... Blah... Blah...

Day #9 and isn't this getting a little bit mundane? I want to make the rest of this journey easier to follow and not turn it into a boring experience, that you can't gain habits and ideas from. So, today I am changing the rest of this journey's format. There will be ONLY meals in Chapter 9. But keep this is mind:

Let me simply and layout my routine...
Every morning (*7-days a week*) I get up early.
And I have 1 bottle of water with lemon in it.
That is all I drink till lunch, it's my semi-morning dry fast. My last water is usually around 6-7 p.m. So, I got dry till 3:30 a.m. so that I can maximize weight loss. During and after my 1 meal. I drink water till bed-time.

At Noon I have my 1 meal, which for the moment I track calories. I do that for 2 reasons: #1. So that I make sure I have a calorie deficiency, so I do loose weight. #2. I make sure there is some substantial nutritional value in my meal.

Then in the afternoon for the remainder of my day I continue to drink water. My goal each day is at least to reach or exceed 100 ounces. I honestly, so far, have not experienced any serious hunger, nothing that noticeable. It is said that thirst can be mistaken for hunger. After I have been drinking so much water now, I agree. I had bad habits in the past, whenever I use to research online, I always enjoyed eating an entire box or Oreo's or any cookies, while I clicked away. To me time passed, and my belly felt satisfied. Well, now I see my health in a different way, and I feel so much better with these newer, smarter habits.

Chapter 9

These Are My **One Meal A Day** Meals

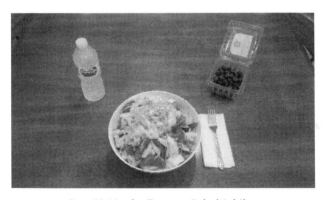

Day #9 Meal – Tomato Salad Jubilee

This was my 1 and only meal today: (12:00 p.m. to 12:30 p.m.)

½ pint of fresh Blueberries (110 calories)
1 Yellow Onion, cut for the salad (115 calories)
3 Vine Tomatoes, cut for the salad (81 calories)
8 oz. Shredded Lettuce, already prepared (25 calories)
½ Large Cucumber, cut for the salad (17 calories)

8 Garlic Cloves, cut for the salad (32 calories)
5 oz. Feta Cheese, for the salad (300 calories)
Olive oil, 1 tbsp. (119 calories)
Apple Cider Vinegar, 2 tbsp. (6 calories)
1 tbsp. of Garlic Powder (32 calories)
Handful of Unsalted Peanuts (200 calories)

My total calorie intake today is: 1,037

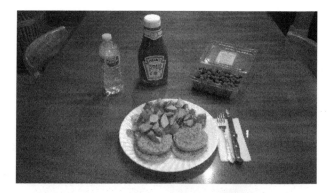

Day #10 Meal – Veggies & Chips

This was my 1 and only meal today: (2:00 p.m. to 2:30 p.m.)

1/2 pint of fresh Blueberries (110 calories)
4 Veggie Burgers, fried, no bread (280 calories)
19 oz. Organic Roasted Red Potatoes, baked (450 calories)
And a bottle of water.

My total calorie intake today is: 840

Day #11 **Today I fasted** straight through to Day #12 I'm finding it so easy to fast now, that I really want to give this a hard push forward. I'm feeling good and I am getting about 7-8 hours' sleep every single night now. So, yes, I will be fasting during my Intermittent Fasting. It'll be a 46-hour fast. I can't to see the results of this. I'm a big guy and I am honestly tired of being so big. I really want to get back to size Medium. I am grateful for this very simple method to get my life back and to be on a much heathier road of habits and my grazing is gone. I honestly don't have any desire for constant or any snacking. And my snacking habits were bad. Today I drank water all day exceeding 100 oz. and I had 5 garlic cloves between 2-3 p.m. for no other reason than to have something. Each clove is 4 calories.

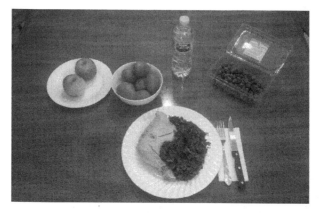

Day #11 Meal – Chicken Tator Popeye

This was my 1 and only meal today: (2:05 p.m. to 2:40 p.m.)

1/2 pint of fresh Blueberries (110 calories)
Medium Fresh Chicken Leg Quarter, boiled (350 calories)
16 oz. Yellow Skinned Potatoes, boiled (330 calories)
11 oz. Chopped Spinach, boiled (128 calories)
2 Medium Fiji Organic Apples (110 calories)
And a bottle of water.

My total calorie intake today is: 1,028

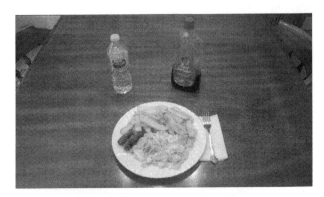

Day #12 Meal – Steak Fries & Scrambled Eggs

This was my 1 and only meal today: (2:00 p.m. to 2:20 p.m.)

5 Lg Scrambled Eggs, fried (450 calories)
6 oz of Steak Fries, 34 pieces, baked (240 calories)
3 Sausage Links, fried (150 calories)
2 tablespoons of Maple Syrup (104 calories)
And a bottle of water.

My total calorie intake today is: 944

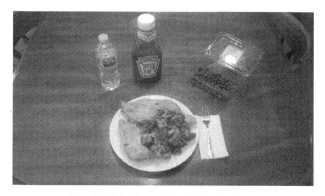

Day #13 Meal – Chicken Bacoli-Berry

This was my 1 and only meal today: (1:00 p.m. to 1:25 p.m.)

1/2 pint of fresh Blueberries (110 calories)
2 Medium Fresh Chicken Leg Quarter, boiled (600 calories)
10.8 oz. Broccoli Florets, boiled (100 calories)
And a bottle of water.

My total calorie intake today is: 820

AWESOME!!! All this hard work is paying off. I have changed a whole bunch of things in my life. I now weigh myself in my bathroom, because I am spending more time in their taking care of my face. LOL... That didn't make sense. What I am doing is exfoliating my facing skin every morning and every evening. Then I am applying with a cotton ball, Organic Apple Cider Vinegar (with the Mother). This is the unpasteurized, made with natural ingredients. It clear pimples, spots and it clears away dead skin. Usually after the 7th day you begin to really see a difference.

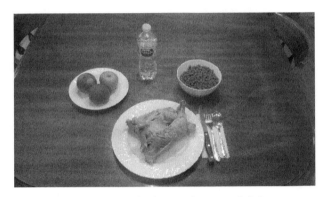

Day #14 Meal – Chicken with Broccoli & Peas

This was my 1 and only meal today: (1:00 p.m. to 1:30 p.m.)

2+ Medium Fresh Chicken Leg Quarter, boiled (600 calories)
12 oz. Sweet Peas, boiled (280 calories)
2 Medium Fiji Organic Apples (110 calories)
1 Medium Tomato (18 calories)
8 Individual Unsalted Peanuts, each are 11 (88 calories)
And a bottle of water.

My total calorie intake today is: 1,006

Day #15 **Today I fasted** straight through to Day #16 I'm finding it so easy to fast now, hunger isn't even an issue. I know, I still have enough for my body to eat off for energy. Ketosis is truly in full effect here. This week I will fast Monday, Wednesday and Friday just to give my weight loss a push and to stay on Ketosis just a bit more. Kind of an after thought. (1:15 p.m. to 1:00 pm) On the days I fast straight through, I will eat 3 small *Organic Fiji Apples* with a sprinkle of cinnamon. Each apple is 55 calories and with a little bit of cinnamon, there won't be 180 calories total.

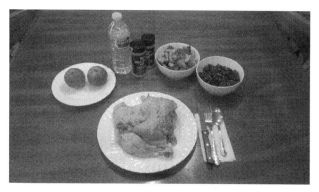

Day #16 Meal – Chicken and Green Veges

This was my 1 and only meal today: (1:10 p.m. to 1:45 p.m.)

2 Medium Fresh Chicken Leg Quarter, boiled (600 calories)
10.8 oz. Broccoli Florets, boiled (100 calories)
11 oz. Chopped Spinach, boiled (128 calories)
2 Medium Fiji Organic Apples (110 calories)
And a bottle of water.

My total calorie intake today is: 938

Day #17 **Today I fasted** straight through to Day #18 I'm finding it so easy to fast now, hunger isn't even an issue. Today I only had an 8 oz. Sweet Potato with 4 Garlic Cloves. Just a little only 200 calories. (12:00 p.m. to 12:25 p.m.) I feel content but not hungry. This has been a fantastic day of energy and inspiration.

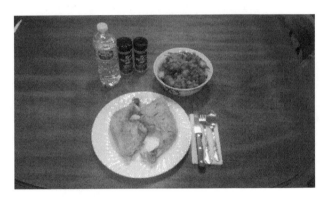

Day #18 Meal – Chicken and Loads of Veges

This was my 1 and only meal today: (2:00 p.m. to 2:30 p.m.)

2 Medium Fresh Chicken Leg Quarter, boiled (600 calories)
12 oz. Sweet Peas and Carrots, boiled (200 calories)
12 oz. Brussel Sprouts, boiled (140 calories)
And a bottle of water.

My total calorie intake today is: 940

Day #19 **Today I fasted** straight through to Day #20 I'm finding it so easy to fast now, hunger isn't even an issue. I feel fantastic and I keep losing weight and yes, I am drinking lots of water. Keep in mind, on the days I skip my one and only meal, get at least 200 calories of food at least in the middle of the day.

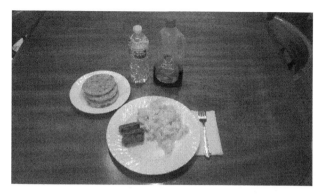

Day #20 Meal – Waffle, 5 Eggs and Sausage

This was my 1 and only meal today: (1:00 p.m. to 1:15 p.m.)

5 Lg Scrambled Eggs, fried (450 calories)
3 Sausage Links, fried (150 calories)
2 tablespoons of Maple Syrup (104 calories)
3 Eggo Chocolate Chip Waffles, toasted (300)
And a bottle of water.

My total calorie intake today is: 994

Today is Day #21 - WEIGH IN !!!! and it looks Fantastic !!!

This is AWESOME!! Progress in this OMAD plan is mind-boggling. I am very committed to it, I never ever cheat, not all, not even a spoon full or just a bite.

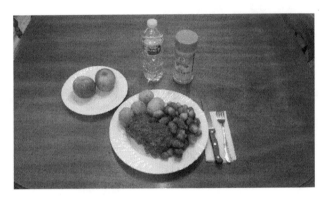

Day #21 Meal – Homemade Meatloaf Delight

This was my 1 and only meal today: (1:00 p.m. to 1:00 p.m.)

8 oz. Homemade Meatloaf, baked (463 calories)
8 oz. Klondike Goldust Baby Potatoes, boiled (165 calories)
12 oz. Brussel Sprouts, boiled (140 calories)
2 Medium Fiji Organic Apples (110 calories)
And a bottle of water.

My total calorie intake today is: 878

Day #22 **Today I fasted** straight through to Day #23 I'm finding it so easy to fast now, hunger isn't even an issue.

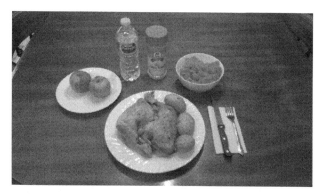

Day #23 Meal – Chicken, Potato and Carrot

This was my 1 and only meal today: (12:20 p.m. to 12:45 p.m.)

2 Medium Fresh Chicken Leg Quarter, boiled (600 calories)
8 oz. Klondike Goldust Baby Potatoes, boiled (165 calories)
8 oz. Crinkle Cut Carrots, boiled (95 calories)
2 Medium Fiji Organic Apples (110 calories)
And a bottle of water.

My total calorie intake today is: 970

Day #24 **Today I fasted** straight through to Day #25 I'm finding it so easy to fast now, hunger isn't even an issue.

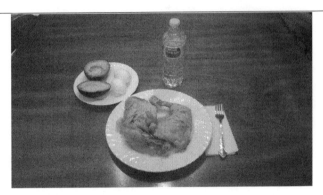

Day #25 Meal – Chicken Avocado

This was my 1 and only meal today: (12:20 p.m. to 12:45 p.m.)

2 Medium Fresh Chicken Leg Quarter, boiled (600 calories)
1 Fresh Avocado (234 calories)
3 Large Hard-Boiled Eggs (234 calories)
And a bottle of water.

My total calorie intake today is: 1,068

Day #26 and Day #27 **I fasted** straight through to Day #28 I'm finding it so easy to fast now, hunger isn't even an issue. I had midday 2-300 calorie snacks and that's it. Basically, I ate Avocado's and Hard-Boiled Eggs.

Day #28 Meal – Chicken and Eggs, Sprouts

This was my 1 and only meal today: (12:00 p.m. to 12:00 p.m.)

2 Medium Fresh Chicken Leg Quarter, boiled (600 calories)
12 oz. Brussel Sprouts, boiled (140 calories)
4 Large Hard-Boiled Eggs (312 calories)

And a bottle of water.

My total calorie intake today is: 1,052

Day #29 **I dry fasted** straight through to Day #30 I'm finding it so easy to fast now, hunger isn't even an issue. I am so excited and thrilled seeing so much progress.

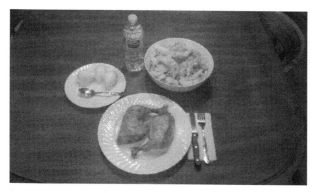

Day #30 Meal – Chicken and Salad and Eggs

This was my 1 and only meal today: (1:25 p.m. to 1:55 p.m.)

2 Medium Fresh Chicken Leg Quarter, boiled (600 calories)
12 oz. Tossed Salad, fresh (140 calories)
3 Large Hard-Boiled Eggs (234 calories)
Small ½ handful of unsalted peanuts (125)
And a bottle of water.

My total calorie intake today is: 1,099

Day #31 **I fasted** straight through to Day #32. I had midday 2-300 calorie snacks and that's it. Basically, I ate Avocado's and Hard-Boiled Eggs.

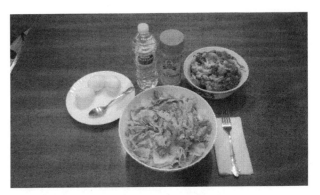

Day #32 Meal – Grilled Chicken Salad, Broccoli and Eggs

This was my 1 and only meal today: (1:00 p.m. to 1:00 p.m.)

12 oz. Tossed Salad, fresh (140 calories)
7 oz. Grilled Chicken Pieces (500 calories)
12 oz. Broccoli Florets, boiled (120 calories)
3 Large Hard-Boiled Eggs (234 calories)
And a bottle of water.

My total calorie intake today is: 1,012

Day #33 **I fasted** straight through to Day #34. I had midday 2-300 calorie snacks and that's it. Basically, I ate Avocado's and Hard-Boiled Eggs.

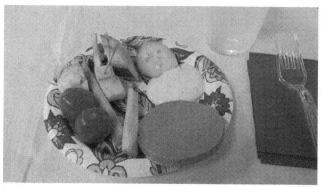

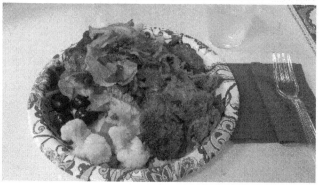

Meal #34 – Appetizer and Pulled Beef at a Party

Today I went to my friend, Marie's birthday party. I have no clue about the calories, I ate in moderation and I focused on vegetables and salad the most and I always only drink water. I figured I have been on this so long is shouldn't affect my weight. I know what to stay away from and what is really healthy to eat.

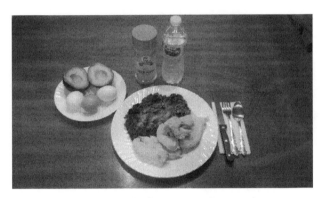

Meal #35 – Chicken Breast & Spinach

This was my 1 and only meal today: (11:35 p.m. to 12:00 p.m.)

15 oz. Boneless Chicken Strips, boiled (500 calories)
12 oz. Chopped Spinach, boiled (140 calories)
1 Raw Avocado, fresh (234 calories)
3 Large Hard-Boiled Eggs (234 calories)
And a bottle of water.

My total calorie intake today is: 1,108

Day #36 **I fasted** straight through to Day #37. I had midday 2-300 calorie snacks and that's it. Basically, I ate Avocado's and 3 Hard-Boiled Eggs.

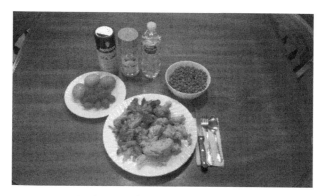

Meal #37 – Chicken and Vegetables

This was my 1 and only meal today: (12:00 p.m. to 12:00 p.m.)

15 oz. Boneless Chicken Strips, boiled (440 calories)
12 oz. Broccoli Florets, boiled (120 calories)
6 oz. Sweet Peas, boiled (140 calories)
1 Medium Hard-Boiled Organic Eggs (60 calories)
7 Cherry Tomatoes, Fresh (15 calories)
And a bottle of water.

My total calorie intake today is: 775
(This meal started out large 1,114 calories, I was full, so I changed it.)

Day #38 **I fasted** straight through to Day #39. I had midday 2-300 calorie snacks and that's it. Basically, I ate Avocado's and 3 Hard-Boiled Eggs.

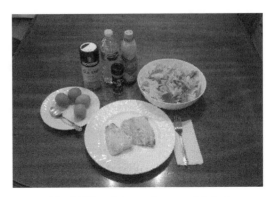

Meal #39 – Salmon Eggs and Salad

This was my 1 and only meal today: (11:50 p.m. to 12:15 p.m.)

8 oz. Salomon, microwaved (260 calories)
12 oz. Lettuce Salad, fresh (60 calories)
5 Medium Hard-Boiled Organic Eggs (300 calories)

And a bottle of water.

My total calorie intake today is: 620

Day #40 **I fasted** straight through to Day #41. I had midday 3-400 calorie healthy snacks and that's it. Basically, I ate an Avocado and 3 Hard-Boiled Eggs.

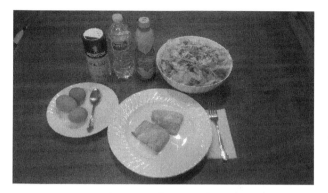

Meal #41 – Salmon and Salad

This was my 1 and only meal today: (12:00 p.m. to 12:00 p.m.)

8 oz. Salomon (wild caught), microwaved (260 calories)
12 oz. Lettuce Salad, fresh (60 calories)
5 oz. Super Blend added to Salad, fresh (50 calories)
3 Medium Hard-Boiled Organic Eggs (180 calories)
And a bottle of water.

My total calorie intake today is: 550 (this was very filling)

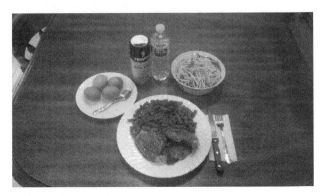

Meal #42 – Chicken BBQ and Eggs

This was my 1 and only meal today: (12:05 p.m. to 12:30 p.m.)

15 oz. Boneless Chicken Strips, boiled (440 calories)
12 oz. Cut Green Beans, boiled (100 calories)
5 oz. Super Blend Mix, fresh (60 calories)
2 Large Hard-Boiled Organic Eggs (120 calories)
And a bottle of water.

My total calorie intake today is: 720 (this too was very filling)

Day #43 **I fasted** straight through to Day #44. I had midday 3-400 calorie healthy snacks and that's it. Basically, I ate an Avocado and 3 Hard-Boiled Eggs.

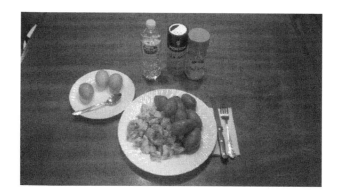

Meal #44 – Chicken w/ Potatoes and Eggs

This was my 1 and only meal today: (12:00 p.m. to 12:00 p.m.)

15 oz. Boneless Chicken Strips, boiled (440 calories)
16 oz. Baby Red Skinned Potatoes, boiled (330 calories)
2 Large Hard-Boiled Organic Eggs (120 calories)
And a bottle of water.

My total calorie intake today is: 890

Day #45 **I fasted** straight through to Day #46. I had midday 3-400 calorie healthy snacks and that's it. Basically, I ate a Pint of Blueberries and 3 Hard-Boiled Eggs.

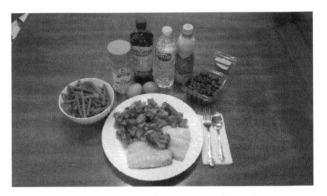

Meal #46 – Salmon Vegetables

This was my 1 and only meal today: (3:30 p.m. to 4:00 p.m.)

8 oz. Salomon (wild caught), microwaved (260 calories)
10 oz. Organic Whole Green Beans, steamed (120 calories)
10 oz. Organic Broccoli Florets, steamed (70 calories)
2 Large Hard-Boiled Organic Eggs (120 calories)
1 Pint of Blueberries, fresh (170 calories)
And a bottle of water.

My total calorie intake today is: 740

Chapter 10

Me Today!

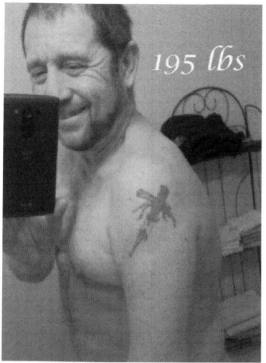

195 lbs

April 2019

This is me NOW! Pictures taken in April 2019

The weight is still off, and I feel absolutely amazing.

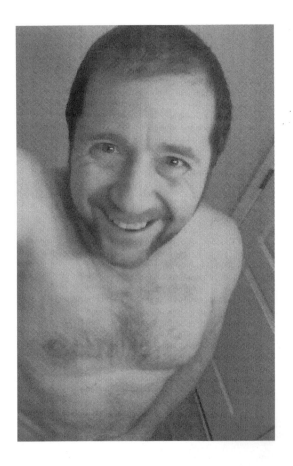

Let me finalize this by saying a lot, so you do know how much this has changed my life. Before I began this, I weighed in at 271 pounds and I was on a lot of medication and I was suffering from my stroke side effects.

NOW, my whole world has changed.

I now weigh in at 195 pounds. I remain on only 1 blood pressure pill by choice, I did that after a conversation with my doctor. Since I am prone to high blood pressure, even though I lost so much weight and don't medically need them; it would be wiser to stay on one to prevent any issues, to be safe. So, I did.

I walk all the time now. In-fact at the time I am writing this, I walk 14-20 miles every other day and I stay focused at a minimum of 10,000 steps a day. Walking has become the saving grace of activity that I believe has played a significant role in my weight loss and my overall optimum health.

My Personal Care Physician (my Doctor) plus my Neurologist plus a DOT Doctor have given me a clean bill of health. I am 100% healed. Meaning I no longer have my stroke side effects at all in my life, period. Plus, I am can function 100% completely normal in all facets of my life. I can even go back to work now. A lot has changed in my life since this journey began, but it is all for the better.

PS. This was all **self-edited by me**, the author, the guy who lost all the weight. I wrote this while I was actually going through the day to day experience of it, one day hoping to share it. Since I got my clean bill of health, I was even more excited to share it. I hope this book has been helpful to you. I continue to research and stay healthy. I will be writing more books as my health only gets better.

Made in the USA
Las Vegas, NV
02 August 2022

52577227R00028